Portrait of
Indifference

Portrait of Indifference

A Comparative Materia Medica

Supplement to
Portraits of
Homoeopathic
Medicines
Volume Two

North Atlantic Books
Wehawken Book Company
Homeopathic Educational Services

Catherine R. Coulter

Portrait of Indifference
A supplement to *Portraits of Homoeopathic Medicines,*
Volume Two

Copyright © 1989 by Catherine R. Coulter

ISBN 1–55643–077–9

Publishers' Addresses:

> North Atlantic Books
> 2800 Woolsey Street
> Berkeley, California 94705
>
> Homeopathic Educational Services
> 2124 Kittredge Street
> Berkeley, California 94704
>
> Wehawken Book Company
> 4221 45th Street N.W.
> Washington, D.C. 20016

Cover and book design by Paula Morrison
Typeset in Garamond by Classic Typography

Portrait of Indifference is sponsored by the Society for the Study of Native Arts and Sciences, a nonprofit educational corporation whose goals are to develop an ecological and crosscultural perspective linking various scientific, social, and artistic fields; to nurture a holistic view of arts, sciences, humanities, and healing; and to publish and distribute literature on the relationship of mind, body, and nature.

Contents

Indifference

> Indifference: "Lack of feeling for or against anything: apathy; lack of sufficient importance to constitute a difference; not easily interested or moved; neither good nor bad, desirable nor undesirable."

The Nature of Indifference

This mental state, defined by Webster mainly in negative terms to portray an emotional void, is actually a highly complex emotion, full of substance and fraught with inner tension. Its manifestations differ in the various constitutional types and according to the causes from which it originates.

For instance, in *Phosphorus* indifference often takes the form of unresponsiveness, in *Lycopodium* of detachment, in *Sulphur* of egocentricity, in *Natrum muriaticum* of self-denial, in *Sepia* of lack of interest, in *Lachesis* of "switching off," and so forth.

Sometimes the indifference appears innate (*Lycopodium*), sometimes acquired (*Phosphorus, Phosphoric acid*), sometimes assiduously cultivated (*Natrum muriaticum, Staphysagria*), sometimes a blend of the above (*Sepia*).

In its purest form, indifference is a sickness arising from total physical collapse or mental shock, with no strength to care, and is addressed by such remedies as *Phosphoric acid* and *Carbo vegetabilis*. But sometimes it is part of a *curative process*—offering the vulnerable individual a way to find emotional equilibrium and assisting him to become disengaged from unendurable reality.

In these cases the physician will administer medium instead of high potencies so as not to disturb the defence mechanisms at work. For the action of the homoeopathic remedy is paradoxical: the one that can dispel an unhealthy indifference can sustain and encourage a curative one.

The physician further learns to distinguish a true emptiness from one which masks an underlying vulnerability or obsession. And this latter state can, in turn, be subdivided into healthy versus unhealthy masking indifference—all of which forms will be examined below.

However, sustained indifference, even when curative, is often unnatural. Feeling, caring, enjoying, relating, being moved by interest or curiosity, are all integral to being human, and a true indifference, in the sense of emotional stasis, denies a vital aspect of the human experience. Even the "healing" (or "protective") indifference, taking the form of self-renunciation or self-deprivation, entails a certain degree of withdrawal from life. And the individual who remains too long in an emotional void, lacking positive feelings, risks replenishing the vacuum with negative ones. Forestalling this evil by extricating the patient from his slough of indifference and restoring him to a fuller state of existence becomes the physician's prime objective.

Yet another species of indifference is not a rejection of life, but only a rejection of overly powerful and uncontrolled emotions which endanger one's serenity. It is the calm after an emotional storm, emerging when pain and bitterness have been exhausted, emotional injury and disappointment overcome, rancour and resentment dispersed. The patient has progressed beyond the subversive anger that tends to turn against him, beyond "extreme loathing of life" (Hahnemann—*Sepia*), and has arrived instead at an indifference that offers a way of confronting harrowing emotional ambiguities and softening rigidities of personality without risking a fracture. The task of the homoeopathic remedies may often be to help the patient arrive at this highly desirable state of poise and serenity.

The term "indifference" thus covers a range of functions, both curative and masking, emotions both healthy and unhealthy, and manifestations both desirable and undesirable—meaning, in homoeopathy, that we have a large assortment of possible medicines. Apart from *Phosphoric acid,* the newest member of our portrait gallery, the following pages touch primarily upon the finer shadings of several remedies already discussed in these *Portraits.*

This selection merely reflects the author's own observations and experience with cases exhibiting the emotional state called "indifference" and is not meant to exclude such remedies as *China, Platina, Lilium tigrinum,* and dozens of others which have also been found to benefit patients in whom indifference is a prominent symptom.

Genuine Indifference Resulting from Physical Ailments or Mental Shock

A genuine indifference, in the sense of true emotional emptiness, can be provoked by such acute physical ailments as influenza, pneumonia, mononucleosis, malaria, typhoid, and others. The patient is left too feeble to muster a mental or emotional response.

Carbo vegetabilis comes first to mind for the utter indifference accompanying the state of collapse following a severe illness. The patient is aware of his surroundings but "hears everything without feeling pleasantly or unpleasantly, and without thinking of it" (Hering). He cannot "whip himself into activity or rouse a desire to do anything . . . [and is] unable to perceive or feel the impressions that circumstances ought to arouse" (Kent). These mental symptoms reflect one aspect of the well-attested *Carbo vegetabilis* "sluggishness" (Kent).

But overall this polychrest suffers from a paucity of idiosyncratic or sharply delineated psychological traits. In addition to its picture of indifference and mental sluggishness, the sketchy mental picture of this important remedy is made up principally of variations on Hering's "memory feeble or temporarily lost . . . with a tendency to fixed ideas; mental confusion making thinking difficult" and Hahnemann's "out of humor, great irritability, peevishness; impatient after angry outburst of temper."

Another commonly prescribed medicine for indifference after an exhausting illness (influenza in particular) is *Gelsemium.* Here the mental "dullness, listlessness, and languor" (Boericke) correspond to the patient's physical picture of droopy eyelids, heavy limbs, and complete absence of energy. And, in a perhaps fanciful extension of the Law of Similars, the state of both mind and body are reminiscent of the torpid, sultry languor induced by the intoxicating perfume of the yellow jasmine from which the remedy derives.

Psorinum should also be considered for indifference arising from lowered vitality and lingering weakness in a patient never fully recovered from some previous illness—a "never *cared* since" syndrome which parallels the "never well since" syndrome discussed in an earlier chapter.

Phosphoric acid is another viable candidate for total indifference to his surroundings. Although Boericke says of it, "mental debility comes first, followed later by the physical," many physicians find it uesful in cases of indifference following a debilitating physical illness, where the patient simply has *too little energy to care.*

Indifference can also result from severe mental *shock*—after a fright or overwhelming sorrow.

The immediate aftermath might call for *Aconite* or *Ignatia.* But once the initial shock has been overcome, *Opium* with its "ailments that originate from fright" (Hering) or *Phosphoric acid,* with its "system [that] has been exposed to the ravages of grief and loss" (Boericke) are frequently resorted to.

Opium's "stupefaction [and] indifference" (Hahnemann) is easily recognized by those familiar with the effects of opium and other opiates ("complains of nothing, wants nothing; tranquil indifference to earthly things": Hahnemann) and requires no further clarifying examples.* But the *Phosphoric acid* indifference that descends on the patient who has undergone the shock of "grief, chagrin, or disappointment in love" (Hering) does call for elaboration.

Like a stone thrown into still waters, after the initial shattering, the emotions spend themselves in a series of ripples of decreasing intensity, and *Phosphoric acid* is a major remedy for these peripheral reverberations. Thus it better fits the second stage of emotional trauma, when acute shock has become a "settled despair" (Boericke) that may take the form of indifference.

The *Phosphoric acid* patient is quiet and seemingly unperturbed. Although he might appear absorbed, in reality no feelings or sensations smolder beneath the surface ("no howling emptiness inside," as one patient put it). He is adverse to conversation and unable to react appropriately ("speaks little and answers unwillingly the questions put to him": Hahnemann)—not because he is sullen or out of humor (although he may "look very ill-humored and sullen": Hahnemann), but from a sense of futility. No comment is adequate to the trauma he is undergoing or has undergone, and no one who has not experienced a similar grief can understand it. He does not permit himself to feel, lest he reopen old wounds and rekindle the former pain. He will dutifully go through the required motions of living but appears abstracted—almost in a dream. Or he will sit numb and dazed, staring vacantly into space.

He might tell himself to clean the house, work in the garden, or visit a friend, but then appends, "Why bother? Why pretend to care? Nothing matters any more . . ." In extreme cases he takes to his bed, lying motionless, "like a log, utterly regardless of his surroundings" (H.C. Allen), and unwilling to be disturbed.

---

*However, the reader is reminded of the remedy's unique role in that extreme case of indifference—unconsciousness from a severe head injury or other such cause (secondarily, *Belladonna* and *Helleborus*).

Phosphoric acid, however, may also be indicated for the polar opposite of indifference—the *overt* forms of grieving where the patient is visibly torn asunder, uncontrolled and frantic ("hysteria": Hering; "restlessness . . . weeping . . . hurried talking": Hahnemann).

A woman of fifty, diagnosed several years earlier with multiple sclerosis, suddenly realized that her condition was incurable. She had been valiantly ignoring it and trying to live normally, but her progressive physical disability now caused her continually to trip and fall. In the last few months she had gone from a cane to a walker, and was now confined to a wheelchair. Her back hurt continuously; at night she had severe tearing pains in the legs; she had neither bowel nor urinary control; and her clumsy fingers could not open jars or bottles, or even hold objects without dropping them. Her tongue, moreover, was so thick and inagile that she sounded inebriated when she spoke.

Hence she had totally lost her composure and came to the physician sobbing in terror and despair.

Ignatia was initially prescribed for her hysteria, and several other remedies were tried, but the case was really turned around by *Phosphoric acid* 200C (in weekly doses for a month) with its two rather colorless supporting symptoms: "better for warmth of bed and warm food" (Hering).

Today, ten years later, the patient has not been cured of her degenerative disease but has very definitely improved. She can walk with only occasional use of a cane, has nearly full control of her bowels and urine, talks normally, and has recovered more than eighty percent of her manual dexterity. She receives constitutional remedies at least monthly to maintain her improvement, and if she relapses into overt fear and hopelessness, *Phosphoric acid* invariably comes to the rescue.

Worth mentioning, in connection with this case, is that *Phosphoric acid*, with its "extremities weak and greatly debilitated; tearing pains in joints, bones, and periosteum; stumbles easily and makes mistakes," and *Picric acid* (TNT!), with its "great weakness of the extremities, tired heavy feeling all over body, especially the limbs; acute ascending paralysis" (Boericke), are among the half-score or so remedies that have proven exceptionally valuable in multiple sclerosis."*

Phosphoric acid is another important homoeopathic remedy (cf. *Carbo vegetabilis,* above) that is not endowed with a well-developed or clearly defined personality. Although possessing a rich and varied collection of physical symptoms, its mental and emotional picture is rather meagre—always overshadowed by the related, and more colorful, *Phosphorus.* Hering has summarized the *Phosphoric acid* personality in a few key traits: "unwilling to speak; listless, apathetic; *remarkably indifferent to everything in life . . .* weak memory; loss of ideas; weakness of mind; cannot collect thoughts; cannot find the right word when talking; answers reluctantly and slowly, or shortly and incorrectly." Later textbooks of *materia medica* merely reiterate this picture, or elaborate on it, and the prescriber must rely largely on the physical symptoms and supporting modalities.

Yet, in its power to dispel the indifference resulting from despondency, negativity, lack of interest, or emotional emptiness, to restore the physically exhausted or emotionally depleted patient's vitality and ability to care; also in its capacity to enable the despairing patient to acquire a *saving* indifference, and the stoical one to sustain his mental equilibrium through mental and emotional strain— *Phosphoric acid* has earned its rightful place among the homoeopathic polychrests.

---

*Others are: *Natrum muriaticum, Plumbum, Causticum, Staphysagria, Nux vomica, Phosphorus, Gelsemium,* and *Ignatia.* The patient will usually gravitate among several of these during the always lengthy course of treatment.

The Masking Indifference

Often the indifference is not genuine but merely feigned—a sheath concealing some underlying drive, fear, or vulnerability. The aim is not to deceive. The mask of indifference helps preserve self-control and maintain emotional stability; it serves to contain an otherwise consuming emotion. It also signals to others that this reserve should not be violated but be respected.

Phosphoric acid plays a major role in all these instances.

A representative case was the middle-aged man suffering from arthritic pains of recent onset who, with the noblest intentions in the world, could scarcely tolerate the chronic infidelities of his attractive young wife. His love for her and their two young children, together with his innate stoicism, enabled him to conceal his pain behind a mask of indifference, and his calm disposition, seemingly incapable of rancour, helped him appear unperturbed. Only his sorrowful, pleading eyes—those of a dog gazing imploringly at his master and unable to express his pain—betrayed his true feelings. Although he forgave his wife in his heart and appeared indifferent to her behavior, his body possessed a will of its own. Expressing its grief through the pain in its joints, it refused to allow him to ignore the repeated injuries to his psyche.

Being closely related chemically to *Phosphorus, Phosphoric acid* has the same affinity for the bones and joints—with "tearing," "burning," "boring," "digging," or "cramping" pains—and this remedy was prescribed (in medium potencies) with gratifying results. The physical pain vanished, and even the emotional trauma became more tolerable.

Admittedly, other homoeopathic remedies are available to assist patients who conceal their injuries under a cloak of indifference, but whose unforgiving and unforgetting body develops pathology in consequence. *Natrum muriaticum* is a prime example—hiding his sorrow under a beaming smile so as not to burden others with his interminable difficulties ("No, nothing's the matter . . . Yes, I'm perfectly fine!'') or maintaining a stoic front and stiff upper lip to prevent his feelings from becoming too real.

Prominent here, too, is *Staphysagria*—whose masking indifference conceals even from himself the emotional origins of his bursitis, rheumatism, sciatica, tendonitis, or whatever.

Sometimes, in fact, the patient recognizes the emotional basis of his illness only in hindsight—after *Staphysagria* has been successfully prescribed and helped to cure his physical condition.

A typical case was the woman with a persistent sciatica which resisted all pain-killers. After trying every conceivable medical test, including a CAT scan, she eventually turned for help to homoeopathy. At first she was treated with such conventional sciatica remedies as *Rhus toxicondendron, Hypericum,* and *Colocynthis,* but when these proved unavailing, the physician inquired more closely about her family. Underlying her condition, as it turned out, was anger at her son's schoolteacher, who was critical of his behavior and insensitive to his needs. She disguised this by a cavalier indifference (''So, she's incompetent. I suppose she cannot help *that.* Anyway, she'll be out of his life after this year!''), but her body did not allow her to suppress this resentment and asserted itself in no uncertain terms until the situation was righted by *Staphysagria.*

Such are the psychic depths addressed by the homoeopathic remedy even without the patient's conscious participation. Without forcing him laboriously to examine the distressing present, or to disinter and relive the traumatic past (in this case, it was the excessive parental criticism the patient had been subjected to in childhood), the simillimum proceeds to disperse their untoward consequences.

Indifference to Everything in Life

''Indifference'' in the Kent *Repertory* has a number of subrubrics. We begin with the one which is broadest in scope—''indifference to everything in life.''

This state is akin to *ennui,* that mental weariness and overall dissatisfaction with life which in former years was regarded as a malady of the leisured class but which today, under conditions of democracy, is shared equally by all.

The patient does not display a Hamlet-like loathing for life out of intellectual *Angst* or ambiguity, nor yet a Werther-like *tedium vitae* out of sorrow or despair, with active desire for death; his attitude is more *defeatist*, his mood is calm, but his outlook is somber.

For this condition *Phosphoric acid* is a homoeopathic mainstay. It befits the patient with *complete* lack of interest in his surroundings. Even when young, he is so fatigued in spirit, so firmly convinced that pleasure, success, affection, and excitement are not for him, that he has ceased striving for happiness or meaning in life.

It is not a sense of grievance that deprives him of responsiveness but rather a settled discouragement and demoralization—a dispirited reaction to his environment. He displays no urgency, no desire for accomplishment, no impatience to overcome his mental stagnation—to move out of his emotional limbo. "I need time to remain ill . . . I haven't the energy to start getting well . . . I have to stay in this apathetic state a while longer . . . Please don't force me!"—are his more typical supplications; and "I don't want *any* of your remedies. I *refuse* to be potentized!"—a more unusual one.

A man of the church, who had returned weak and depressed from a tour of the Third World in an official capacity, was loath to resume his parish duties. While the diarrhoea he had contracted in Africa was debilitating enough, something more subtle and profound than any physical ailment had transpired during his trip. Witnessing so much poverty, illness, starvation, and suffering in his enfeebled state had undermined his faith, and he was now quite indifferent to the spiritual welfare of his American flock. He saw no point in continuing his mission on earth. He had, in short, given up: "I feel that I have passed the summit of life; from now on the path goes only downhill."

The minister's uncharacteristic, but now engrained, indifference was so startling that a friend recommended that he try homoeopathy. On the basis of his continuing diarrhoea (prominent in *Phosphoric acid*), and also by virtue of the modality "worse when walking out of doors, better from sitting in the house" (Hahnemann), one of the remedy's few idiosyncratic symptoms, it was prescribed in the 1M potency.

The effect was spectacular! It not only restored the clergyman's former optimism and happy disposition but accomplished the more formidable task of renewing his faith in an ultimately merciful (even if His ways are not always comprehensible) Deity.

The *Phosphorus* "indifference to everything in life" presents an even more striking contrast to the type's usual liveliness or *joie de vivre.* Sometimes his lack of response reflects an overall *satiety* with life's pleasures, after having burnt the candle at both ends— and in the middle. At other times the "strange, rare, and peculiar" aspect is the sudden loss of his former attractive enthusiasms.

A homoeopathic physician in his mid-thirties who was relatively new to the trade suddenly lost all interest in life—including family, friends, hobbies, even (difficult to believe!) his profession. His former ebullience and eagerness to follow the homoeopathic method had turned into a profound despondency ("the whole world seems dreadful to him; only weeping relieves him": Hahnemann) and was later moderated to a less alarming listlessness ("afterwards total apathy": Hahnemann). When he finally turned to a colleague for assistance, the latter had no difficulty arriving at the root of the problem.

Some years earlier this fledgling doctor had been converted to homoeopathy by one of those energetic and charismatic leaders periodically spawned by this movement, who set themselves up as more than mere teachers—rather as "masters" or "gurus"—and thereupon develop a strong and devoted following.

For a few years this patient had been the favorite son, a privileged position which sustained him in his studies and his work. But when he was duly superseded by a younger disciple, the light of his enthusiasm dimmed and was finally extinguished altogether. He no longer had the heart to seek the company of his former colleagues, or even to practice homoeopathy, and became quite indifferent to life.

Phosphorus is an enthusiast and, like many enthusiasts, requires an outside force to nourish and sustain his interest (the *Phosphorus* personality, we recall, may lack a clearly defined core or sense of identity), and in these cases his enthusiasm is a weakness rather than a strength. When this nourishing force withdraws, he is lost and empty, unable to function on his own. He then laments the unsubstantiated promises, which are no less meaningful to him for being largely tacit, and feels rejected and bereft. Furthermore, because it is an "outside" force that he has never fully understood, he is confronted with the pain of disillusionment in a God (who "passeth human understanding") that has failed. Such was this patient's predicament.*

He had dosed himself with *Aurum metallicum, Ignatia, Natrum muriaticum,* and other remedies, but he started slowly to pull out of his debilitating mental state only when *Phosphorus* was prescribed—largely on the contrast between his present indifference and his former strong enthusiasm. He eventually resumed his former practice—in a quieter mode but this time with truer inner strength.

Natrum muriaticum can be equally indifferent to life after some painful disillusionment or loss of enthusiasm but has another mode of reaction. He seldom abandons completely any activity involving an element of duty and thus, despite his current apathy, joylessly goes through the motions of what was once meaningful. Hence his

---

*Admittedly, this is the dilemma of any enthusiast, whatever the constitutional type (cf. *Ignatia* in love). Because he cannot nourish himself, he demands of his idol ever greater feats of performance (enthusiasm leeches even as it supports), and all but the most deft leaders of men are hence placed in the precarious, not to say false, position of having to extend themselves beyond their natural capacities in order to satisfy and accommodate their followers.

indifference is burdened with more subliminal anger and resentment than that of *Phosphorus, Phosphoric acid,* or *Carbo vegetabilis.*

However, it is rarely maintained with any consistency. Rather it alternates with spells of diligence, animation, and resurging enthusiasm, and this all contributes to the type's well-known mood swings and sudden reversals of taste and opinion.

Although *Natrum muriaticum* might be genuinely indifferent to his own life or welfare, he is not indifferent to death. While perhaps welcoming it in the abstract, he cannot be apathetic about leaving the world improperly attended to. Who will set things right once he has departed? Hence he must stay around—at least until someone equally farseeing and responsible materializes to take over his important duties. What is more, when he does recover from a debilitating indifference, he embraces life with the eagerness appropriate to one miraculously vouchsafed another opportunity of assisting a world in travail.

Lycopodium presents quite another picture of "indifference to the highest degree . . . insensibility to external impressions" (Hahnemann). Ever sceptical of emotion and both relativistic and ambivalent in his perception of the world, his apathy seldom proceeds from lost enthusiasm but is rather an offshoot of his innate detachment. He both instinctively and on principle repudiates whatever jeopardizes this detachment: any enthusiasm, eagerness, or too-strong emotion.

A case emblematic of *Lycopodium*'s principled reluctance to betray enthusiasm was the lady gardener whose growing indifference to life had been exacerbated by a mid-life depression. When challenged by a friend to react to a beautiful bed of geraniums, she replied: "I don't find this flower bed the least bit interesting. But perhaps the fault lies in the geraniums themselves and not in my own apathy. Uninspiring flowers at best, they do not grip the attention of even the healthiest individuals."

This *Lycopodium* characteristic is not easily analyzed but is best appreciated in context. Another instance is his way of reacting to another's excited concern with a cool "Does it really matter?" Indeed, in cosmic terms, the event might not really matter, but it was not seen that way until *Lycopodium* placed it in perspective.

Or, when told that some undertaking is bound to be "unforgettable," *Lycopodium* may remark wryly, "That is certainly possible!" The implication, of course, is that the experience may well match the enthusiast's expectations, but not necessarily in the way desired.

Such laconic, even-tempered scepticism could be viewed, charitably, as reluctance to take too seriously his own or another's feelings—a healthy characteristic when not accompanied by emotional withdrawal. Those less partial to the typical *Lycopodium* aloofness ascribe this "indifference" to an unyielding desire for psychological mastery.

In *Calcarea carbonica,* "indifference to everything in life" carries a note of *resignation.*

In sickness this can appear as "indifference about his recovery" (Kent) with loss of all desire to fight illness.* In health he may refuse to worry about the morrow: "What will be, will be," states he with oriental fatalism. "Sufficient unto the day are the problems thereof."

Thus he resists the modern tempo of haste and urgency and handles all conflicts and ambiguities through a placid indifference. Tracing back through the case history, the physician may find indifference rooted in disappointment that some anticipated event did not occur, some long-awaited change never came to pass. The patient has relinquished hope and become indifferent so as not to be disappointed a second time.

It is not only older persons, who may have outlived the need for passion and intensity in their lives, who suffer from phlegmatism

---

*If there has been much physical pain and suffering, the remedy is often *Arsenicum album* ("careless about approaching death, neither hopes nor wishes to recover": Hahnemann).

and inertia, but younger ones as well. This state compares with *Sepia's* emotional "stasis" (Farrington), but without the latter's "soured" outlook. *Calcarea* merely exhibits *a preference for rest over motion*— even if (since life is motion) this entails some denial of life itself.

Oblomov, the archetypal *Calcarea carbonica* figure mentioned by us more than once in these *Portraits,* represents this indifference to everything—the man who wishes only to be left in peace. To achieve this he will sacrifice love, friendship, accomplishment, and even self-respect.

This *Calcarea* indifference, that *neither condemns nor condones* the surrounding world, does not repudiate life generally but simply sets little value on his own.

A kind and sensitive, but lonely, *Calcarea* soul suffered from dizziness, constipation, poor sleep, tension in the neck and shoulders, heartburn, and low self-esteem. In her marriage she had long resigned herself to second-class citizenship, and now, with her children grown and gone, she was also suffering the particular loneliness of the "empty nest syndrome." Her life offered no tragedy or trauma, merely stagnation and an unclear picture of how to use her potential. She had withdrawn into her shell and was "indisposed to talking, without being ill-humored" (Hahnemann). Mindful that at times this type can be jogged out of passive indifference only by some external stimulus, the physician, in the full and august majesty of his authority, instructed her to adopt a kitten and two canaries. This mandate, reinforced by a prescription of the potentized oyster shell, accomplished the desired physical improvement.

And there was even some mental improvement, as seen from her remarks a few months later: "Certainly at birth we are dealt a weaker or stronger hand, but I now realize that this does not justify a fatalistic indifference to the game being played. The challenge lies in *how* you play your cards, in scoring as many tricks as you can. A not-too-original discovery, to be sure, but one which in my apathy I never really absorbed until now." She sighed, "I suppose that, with the kitten now fully grown and the canaries singing away contentedly, I shall have to decide how to play *my* hand better. But, oh my! What a daunting prospect!''

The *Staphysagria* "indifference to everything in life" usually follows some injury or insult which the conscious mind is willing to overlook but the implacable physical constitution has no intention of letting go by.

A young woman, temporarily institutionalized for a nervous breakdown, was unable to pass urine without a catheter. She was the picture of indifference, sitting unreactive and unresponsive and staring all day out the window. Her urinary retention, which had commenced in the hospital, immediately suggested *Staphysagria,* and closer questioning revealed the presence of suppressed indignation. Her room had no doorknob on the inside, and she had been furious at the indignity of being so incarcerated. After carrying on about it for two days, her passion was spent, she relapsed into indifference, and had refused, or been unable, to urinate since that time.

Three doses of the remedy in high potency, administered at twelve-hour intervals, released both her urine and her anger. After this outbreak of emotion she became anxious to be released from the hospital and, in consequence, became cooperative and made a speedy recovery.

Sepia and *Sulphur,* two major remedies in this particular sub-rubric, are accorded much coverage in the following sections. Here we need only state that *Sepia*'s overall indifference ("very indifferent to everything: the death of a near relative or some happy occurrence leave her equally unaffected": Hering)—for which a previous trauma or sorrow cannot always be established—often merely reflects a chronic physical lethargy and prostration that renders her incapable of feeling ("lies [indifferent] with her eyes closed": Kent). *Sulphur*'s indifference to everything, on the other hand, usually strikes the physician as a temporary unnatural state in glaring contrast to the individual's customary assertiveness.

Indifference to Pleasure and Money

Indifference to "everything" is less common than indifference to some particular aspect or area of life. This can be a genuine lack of response, or it can indicate some strong feeling or conviction which the patient is combating. In either case it often serves as a guiding symptom.

Of the numerous subrubrics in the Kent *Repertory,* the most intriguing is "indifference to pleasure, [also] to agreeable things."

"Pleasure" here does not mean merely sensual gratification—indulgence in comfort, sexuality, rest, and beauty—although elements of these are naturally present. We speak rather of pleasure in its eighteenth-century acceptation—as a man's *innate* and *legitimate heritage.* Or, to quote from Wordsworth's *Preface to Lyrical Ballads,* "the grand elemental principle [that constitutes] the native and naked dignity of man . . . [and is the means] by which man knows and feels and lives and moves."

This bold assertion places pleasure at the very core of man's self-definition: our very humanity resides in the ability to experience and appreciate pleasure. Indifference to pleasure thus suggests some gross psychic deformity, the negation of some vital human attribute.

The role of *Phosphoric acid* in this particular category is marginal. His indifference to pleasure usually reflects one aspect of his overall emotional emptiness. He cannot respond to pleasurable stimuli because of protracted low-key depression and a low level of energy ("great general weakness": Clarke). Nothing is worth struggling for; he is neither comfortable nor uncomfortable, neither happy nor sad; pleasure is a matter of indifference because life no longer holds out promise or hope.

Phosphoric acid was the middle-aged woman, somewhat overweight, who at night frequently passed large quantities of colorless urine. Her most arresting feature, however, was her attitude. "I feel gray, flat, lifeless, unmotivated, completely uninterested *and* uninteresting. I don't know why I don't sketch any more—I used to enjoy it. I suppose I should take it up again, but—" She shrugged indifferently.

"Don't you enjoy anything at all?" the physician inquired solicitously.

She thought for a long moment. "Not really. I derive a little pleasure from being subtly condescending to my dull neighbors—if that can be considered a legitimate pleasure. But most of the time I can't be bothered to do even that." So saying, she heaved a sigh of regret at lost opportunities.

This was, admittedly, not much to prescribe on in a condition for which many suitable polychrests are available. Still, the physician grabbed at this straw ("indisposed even for pleasant mental work": Hahnemann), and, once on the trail of *Phosphoric acid,* found another symptom to clinch his choice of remedy. The patient could not fall asleep again after her numerous risings to urinate without drinking a few sips of fruit juice. Water, milk, various herb teas, and the like would not serve. She *had* to have fruit juice; otherwise she stayed awake for the rest of the night.

"Desires fruit [and] juicy things" (Kent) is the key to *Phosphoric acid*. This symptom, coupled with the mild diabetes of middle age for which this remedy is frequently indicated, left little doubt as to the curative prescription.

The *Carbo vegetabilis* indifference to pleasure is suggested by Hahnemann's observation, "music which he loves does not affect him."

A case in point was the man with a nondescript lingering cough and faulty digestion. While the physician was searching for some guiding symptom, he volunteered: "I cannot experience any joy in life at all, even in my favorite pastimes. Certainly I feel debilitated from the many stresses on me, but even a passive occupation like watching television gives me no satisfaction whatever—perhaps because of the dreadful commercials!"

"You could set your dial to the non-commercial channels, such as Public Television," the physician suggested. "And leave it there."

"I've already tried that. But I am bored by these 'tasteful' nature shows and the 'intelligent' scientific documentaries. I'm even tired of the impeccably acted British drama serials. I'm simply indifferent to them all!"

Well, he did seem beyond redemption!

For, to this patient the visual and performing arts had been the breath of life. He would describe a good movie as "a religious experience," or a well-acted play as "a mystical revelation." Even a patch of canvas with squiggly lines or some random daubs of color could bring a glistening to his eyes, as he would murmur, "After all, art *is* the only thing in the world worth living for!"

In the very exaggeration of his new attitude, however, lay his homoeopathic redemption. It was so obviously a variation on the *Carbo vegetabilis* indifference to "music which he loves" (Kent) that the physician prescribed this remedy with complete confidence in its success.

Unlike the indifference of *Staphysagria* which, often resulting from some profound injury, leaves him unable to respond even to pleasure ("the most attractive things make no impression on him"' Hahnemann), *Sepia*'s indifference to pleasure ("an absence of all joy . . . no affection for the delightful things of life": Kent) is largely caused by physical fatigue. She is simply too tired.

We recall that the *Sepia* woman, when urged to converse or socialize, may lack the energy even to pull the muscles of her face into a smile, to articulate words, eat, or look and respond appropriately—far less take pleasure in an agreeable social gathering, in the beauties of nature or art, or in the attractive features of an interlocutor.

Her indifference is at times so pervasive that she cannot even *envisage* change and is quite indifferent to the outcome of events. Yet, when her physical lassitude does not correspond in degree to her mental apathy, the physician might detect a subliminal longing to experience pleasure: "Is this the way everyone goes through life?" she laments. "Without happiness? Without any interest in pleasure? What a dreary and dismal thought!"

That the aspiration of this *Sepia* to a fuller and more joyous life is genuine—in contrast to the neurotic type who will not relinquish her misery—is demonstrated by her *transformation* (no other word will do!) when engaged in a vigorous adrenalin-stimulating activity.

Her indifference to pleasurable pursuits may extend also to food. "I simply don't have any appetite whatever" is a common remark.

This state is not to be confused with anorexia (although *Sepia* can be anorexic)—where the patient is actually obsessed by food and deliberately curbs her intake out of pride in her self-control, to demonstrate how little she needs to survive (*Arsenicum*), to punish herself (*Natrum muriaticum*), or out of grief (*Ignatia*). The basis for *Sepia*'s lack of interest in food is often a sluggish digestion that renders all victuals unattractive.

One patient's confusing picture of menopausal depression, frequent hot flashes, and other symptoms had the physician wavering among *Sulphur, Lachesis, Pulsatilla,* and *Sepia.* He finally opted for the latter when she said, "While I am not a great eater at the best of times, lately I have had no interest in food at all. It settles heavily in my stomach and remains lodged there in mute protest. Most trying of all are my routine duties as cook for the household!"

The woman who wants nothing to do with the rituals of nourishing herself or others is very often a *Sepia.*

Sulphur's indifference to the pleasures of the table reflects less a distaste for food than obliviousness to what he eats, when he eats, and even whether he eats, because his mind is occupied with "higher" things.

This type's *lack of interest* in material pleasures differs from the *incapacity* of *Sepia, Phosphoric acid,* or *Carbo vegetabilis* to experience agreeable sensations. It reflects absorption in his own thoughts, with resultant obliviousness to his surroundings ("indifference to external things": Kent). His dreams and imaginings can be so much richer, so much more vivid, than any pleasure offered by the real world that he grows indifferent to the latter. He is not exhausted, merely self-centered.

His indifference to pleasure may also have a philosophical or ideological basis—being rooted more in Thoreau than in any genuine rejection of the world's comforts. For the sake of some higher spirituality he disdains the trivial pursuits, the specious materialism, of contemporary culture. But even the purest and most admirable *Sulphur* ideologue in sincere rebellion against social vanities may possess an Achilles' heel. Although prepared to relinquish most comforts, he will display one particular human weakness—for good wine, or food, or some particular article of attire such as fine leather shoes, silk ties, or a handsome watch. Rakhmetov, hero of Chernyshevskii's novel, *What's To Be Done?* is a perfect example. A revolutionary idealist possessing the typical *Sulphur* streak of asceticism, who rejects every luxury and self-indulgence while striving to build a better world, he still cannot resist the pleasure of smoking very expensive cigars!*

When *Arsenicum album* is indifferent to pleasure, it is usually out of *love for work.* Other pleasures merely distract him from this, the greatest one, and he has no time for them.

Natrum muriaticum, who also senses deeply that luxury and indulgence only distract the high-minded from more significant issues, is more consistent in his indifference to pleasure.

To free himself from "thraldom to the decadent values of a bourgeois society organized for the pursuit of pleasure," as one pa-

---

*The *Sulphur* dandy will betray his constitutional type in a similar way—by some detail which undermines the overall effect. His shirttails protrude out from under his spiffy suit; his expensive and highly polished shoes have holes in the soles, etc.

tient earnestly committed to helping the "underprivileged" put it in all sincerity, he seeks a sort of dignity in *resisting* pleasure. To this constitutional type, who takes a dim view of pleasure in the best of circumstances and who overidentifies with those he is helping, "the native and naked dignity of man" lies not in pleasure but in self-denying renunciation of that which is agreeable.

But *Natrum muriaticum* is an active soul, ever searching out that which defines his humanity, and cannot long remain merely indifferent. The repudiation of pleasure—i.e., denying himself a major avenue of escape from life's hardships—leads inexorably to acceptance of *un*pleasure as an essential feature of his humanity; and he quickly perceives human dignity as residing in the capacity to suffer. Thus his indifference is far from being an emotional void but pulsates with activity and tension, straining to develop into some form of self-punishment or into the particular self-deprivation which so often lies at the root of his actions and reactions.

This is how he boxes himself into the "bleak" mental state for which *Natrum muriaticum* is so well-known.*

However, while indifferent to pleasure, *Natrum muriaticum* can experience *transports of joy*—which is in some ways antagonistic to the calm of pleasure. Usually this transcendent state cannot be long sustained and is soon superseded by a collapse into despondency (also *Phosphorus* and *Lachesis*). This characteristic is one more source of the type's profound mood swings.

Indifference to *money*—not as pleasure *per se* but as a means of obtaining it—requires special consideration. The three remedies coming immediately to mind for the patient who professes this form of indifference are *Sulphur,* followed by *Phosphorus* and *Natrum muriaticum*. Any others trail far behind these three leaders.

Sulphur's indifference to money again proceeds from some ideological conviction. Instead of viewing it as a neutral phenome-

---

*This side of *Natrum muriaticum* has been discussed in Volume I of these *Portraits*.

non, which can be used for good or evil, this constitutional type may despise it for its power to corrupt and may scorn the luxuries, comforts, and pleasures it provides.

This attitude may at times be a mere pose, with the *Sulphur* who professes the greatest indifference in reality respecting money enormously.* But, with his equally high regard for the non-material sphere (ideas, scholarship, learning), *Sulphur* may try to deny his baser instincts. Part of him sincerely yearns for the higher spirituality, and he struggles against his materialistic side (here again, the ''Walden Pond mystique'' of pruning life to the merest necessities). If he cannot actually overcome it, he can at least *talk* as if he has!

Arsenicum album, in contrast, whether generous or parsimonious, well-to-do or impecunious, always respects money and is rarely indifferent to it. How can he be, when he spends so much time worrying about it?

The *Phosphorus* patient who professes indifference to money is usually telling the truth. Possessing little practical sense, he has no particular interest in money and easily lets it slip through his fingers (if a schoolchild or college student, he spends his allowance in the first few days). Even when not simply irresponsible, he refuses to be greatly concerned with money, trusting that—as with the lilies of the field that neither toil nor spin—the Lord will provide.

Lachesis, in contrast, can be equally spendthrift and improvident (we recall the type's addiction to gambling) but is seldom indifferent to money, sensing it too acutely as a symbol of power and guarantor of freedom.

Natrum muriaticum, like *Sulphur,* may also despise money as

---

*Persons who retain in adulthood something of the ''flower child'' mentality of the 1960's are usually strong in *Sulphur;* but in a typical *Sulphur* polarity, many ex-hippies who, with age, turn ultra-materialistic and ultra-fond of the goods of this world are also *Sulphur.* Occasionally this type will admit to being a ''closet materialist.''

the root of evil; or, like *Phosphorus,* he may refuse to preoccupy himself with it. But the tone is different: his indifference seldom works to his own advantage. For the sake of some high-minded principle or noble gesture he will display an exasperating financial naivete.

A divorce lawyer, anxious to promote his clients' welfare, was recounting his professional woes to the homoeopath treating him for burning pains in the stomach. "It is not the aggressive and de- manding clients who give me ulcers. I can handle the ones who are out to wrest every penny from their estranged spouses. But Heaven protect me from the erroneously noble ones who will not stand up for their own interests and who, to avoid hostile feelings or a guilty conscience, constantly undermine my efforts to arrange a fair set- tlement of their property. How can I represent them when they (especially the wives) defend their estranged husbands' interests instead of their own?"

The physician would have liked to have given the frustrated attorney a large vial of *Natrum muriaticum* or *Staphysagria* in the 50M potency for his perverse female clients, but had to content himself with prescribing *Nux vomica* for the man of law himself.

Finally, if dollar bills are consistently found shredded and bleached in the pockets of clothes fresh from the laundry, suggesting a subliminal or principled scorn of money, the possessor of the clothes is bound to have a strong element of *Sulphur* or *Natrum muriaticum* in his constitutional economy.

Money, in its overlapping of work and pleasure, leads to our next topic—indifference to work, professional occupation, or gainful employment.

Indifference to Business and Education

Phosphoric acid will frequently counter a patient's indifference toward his customary work or occupation—the consequence of ex- cessive pressure, among other causes, and usually accompanied by subliminal feelings of failure and defeat.

Manifesting this picture was a clinical psychologist who had suddenly turned apathetic to his profession ("indifference to business affairs": Kent). His most arresting feature was entire loss of his customary good humor and adroitness in dealing with his clients. The psychological defenses which he had formerly succeeded in dismantling, he now found to be insurmountable obstacles.

"To understand people is to get to know their neuroses," he complained. "And my patients' neuroses are nearly always rooted in resentment of their parents and other authority figures, or inability to confront them. *Not* to be angry at one's parents these days argues lack of psychological maturity or, at the least, absence of sensitivity and refinement. As for myself," he continued dispassionately, "I increasingly question the usefulness of my work. Am I deluding myself with an activity of merely pretended importance? Even if, after lengthy treatment, I help one client accept his parents, thousands more out there with the same complexes are waiting to take his place. So what's the point of even trying?"

Such loss of heart and indifference to his vocation was uncharacteristic of this splendid therapist who used to rejoice at every step of his clients' progress. By nature he was quick and articulate, imaginative and inspirational, yet also disciplined and methodical. But neither *Phosphorus* nor *Arsenicum,* his usual constitutional remedies, proved of assistance. The physician then thought of *Phosphoric acid* because of its close chemical relationship to *Phosphorus*—and because there were no contraindications to its selection.

He was not disappointed. When prescribed in the 1M potency, it altered the psychologist's attitude completely, restoring his former self-confidence and dedication to his profession.

Sulphur's indifference to business affairs ("indisposition to work . . . for hours he sits motionless . . . without definite thoughts, though he has many things to do": Hahnemann), is usually caused by some spiritual or existential anxiety and, in extreme cases, is accompanied by the Hobbesian view that life is "nasty, brutish, and short." This attitude, that might encourage him to become a loafer, contrasts with the type's usual happy involvement in gainful employment—be it business, administrative, scholarly, artistic, or even manual pursuits.

Calcarea carbonica's indifference to work may resemble *Sulphur*'s but stems from a deeper stratum of indolence and inertia.

A young man of talent, a senior in a prestigious ivy-league university, was feeling totally indifferent to his future career even while his classmates were energetically preparing for theirs. "I've got a dangerous inheritance," he admitted to his homoeopathic physician. "I am of Russian stock and descend from a family where for generations the men have been mostly supported by the women. I feel there is little your medicines can do for my indifference to matters of career."

He was correct to a degree. He never did become ambitious or truly dedicated to his work, but *Calcarea carbonica* at least encouraged him to get out and hunt for a job—his heredity notwithstanding.

The *Sepia* woman usually enjoys her work, and indifference is therefore due to the by now familiar picture of fatigue. It is often accompanied by a self-deprecating, "I'm not good enough . . . Nobody wants my work anyway . . . So why bother even trying?" etc.

The male may exhibit a similar lack of interest but usually does not denigrate himself. He is just weary of the competitive struggle and longing to retire to the peace and quiet of Maine or Vermont, there to pursue some lower-key interest. *Sepia* in potency has consistently helped women overcome indifference to work by buoying their self-esteem; it also helps men in their professional homestretch pull through the last few years of work before retirement.

Pulsatilla's "indifference to business affairs" (Kent) is characterized by indecisiveness. The mind of this constitutional type is intricate but rarely trenchant because there is no clear reason for choosing one preference, one course of action, over another. This goes hand-in-hand with the conviction that if she (or he) waits long enough, assistance will be forthcoming: "So why should I strain myself?"

Indifference to work can at times be encountered even in *Arsenicum album,* reflecting the "all or nothing" syndrome of this remedy (discussed in that chapter). It contrasts markedly with the customary *Arsenicum* race-horse mentality: nervous, excitable, competitive, determined to lead. The individual becomes apathetic about his work when he can no longer give a peak performance; if he cannot be the best, he prefers to have nothing to do with the field. Hence his indifference conceals an underlying sorrow, regret, even despair, at his loss of capacity.

"No, I am not stupid," commented one *Arsenicum* insomniac whose business was going badly and who wanted—unwisely, as he himself realized—to throw over the whole concern, so apathetic did he feel. "But my work has become meaningless. I feel as though I have been sent down to the minor leagues after playing in the majors. So I prefer to quit altogether."

Thus the *Arsenicum* indifference to work is a perverse reflection of the type's strong drive for excellence and belief in his own competence and distinctiveness—also of his opposition to mediocrity and relentless striving for perfection. In business, as in other spheres, he has the artist's demanding nature, also the artist's tendency to lapse into indifference or despair when his self-imposed goals cannot be attained.

Finally we arrive at the *Natrum muriaticum* indifference which, true to type, presents the most convoluted picture of all.

For this type work is, *inter alia,* a refuge for his thoughts, deflecting them from less pleasant topics. Like *Arsenicum,* he is ever ready to toil in the vineyards with other mortals. Hence, indifference to work (like indifference to pleasure) deprives him of an escape from his inherently bleak outlook or his consuming obsessions.

Always injured by that which he loves best (the champion swimmer becomes allergic to chlorine; the gifted tennis player develops intolerance to the hot sun; the promising painter becomes allergic to turpentine; the fingers of a musician perspire so profusely and peel that he can no longer perform, and so on ad infinitum), *Natrum muriaticum* responds by becoming indifferent to his former professional occupation.* But this quite natural reaction becomes idiosyncratic in the assiduousness and thoroughness with which he carries it through. Cultivation of indifference becomes almost a mission. It is at the least a complex acquired mental state, carefully nurtured to mask the pain of disappointment, quell futile yearnings, and erase the pain of remembered happiness or vanished fulfilment.

Emblematic of this type was the single woman of advancing years, a writer of fiction, who sought homoeopathic aid for a series of complaints, including headaches, a twitching eyelid, itching scalp, and loss of interest in her formerly much-loved vocation. Searching for her remedy the physician encouraged her to talk about her interesting profession. "I have always seen my writing as a long and painful transition from obsession to a healing indifference," she explained, "so that, once I complete a work and arrive at this latter state, I am naturally reluctant to embark again on this torturous course into the realms of disturbing emotion. But I cannot circumvent this stage.** I would like to remain peaceably in my healing indifference, but I am not married, have no independent income, and must earn from my writing. What I would really like is a remedy to counter

---

Natrum muriaticum's indifference to that which he loves best, i.e., his very vocation or raison d'être, differs qualitatively from the "indifference to music which he loves" of *Carbo vegetabilis*. The latter is merely an apathetic response to a pleasurable pursuit.

**It is a truism in literature that one can write *convincingly* only about the emotions one has experienced. In contrast to plot, incident, or dialogue, emotions cannot be invented.

my present *unproductive* indifference without having to relinguish my *protective* one."

The physician pondered this tall order until he understood how fitting it was to the *Natrum muriaticum* mentality to regard artistic creation as a "torturous" transition between obsession and a liberating detachment—instead of a source of pleasurable excitement, self-discovery, intellectual challenge, near-religious ecstasy, or whatever.

The choice of remedy was further confirmed by the two physical symptoms: twitching ("quivering": Kent) of the right upper eyelid and her "impatient scratching of the head" (Hahnemann), and, above all, by the physician's recollection that, despite the patient's asserted pride in her independence and self-sufficiency, all her writings were romances in which the protagonists, after horrendous trials and vicissitudes, inevitably found happiness in one another and "lived happily ever after."

Through her fiction this writer was reworking the reality of her solitary and often lonely existence, to arrive at a state of protective indifference. Her repeated artistic recreation of a reality to which she professed indifference, this sublimation of her emotions, accorded entirely with the *Natrum muriaticum* mentality.*

Not to be forgotten, parenthetically, are those who profess *indifference to criticism of their work*—who seem, in fact, to welcome it—but are really seeking praise.

Arsenicum and *Lycopodium* feign such indifference but cleverly preempt their critics by saying it first, thus protecting their own egos.

Natrum muriaticum and *Calcarea carbonica* at first accept criticism with seeming indifference but then turn defensive, take

---

*The creative process entails reorganizing reality, and in so doing the writer can often free himself of some undesired emotion. But *Natrum muriaticum* can become bogged down in the pain of remembrance, even when striving through artistic creation to relinquish the past. This further exacerbates his misery.

it *too* much to heart, and resent it for years—if not forever.

Phosphorus and *Phosphoric acid,* although anxious to please and liking praise, are often impervious to criticism. While attempting to accommodate their critics, ultimately they proceed along their own free-spirited way.

One patient, who required periodic *Phosphoric acid* as a constitutional remedy for urinary complaints (milky urine, with constant desire), was a man of letters who liked to send his essays to his friends for their evaluation. Since his manner of expressing himself was idiosyncratic, the manuscripts came back drenched in red ink. His friends marvelled at his sanguine attitude under the circumstance and his good-humored attempts to adapt his style to his critics' requirements. Then, one day, in a fit of exasperation, he exclaimed: "When I send out my prose for comment, what I want is positive feedback on my ideas, not criticism of my style. The rules of grammar and punctuation are for foreigners and illiterates, not for me. English is *my* language, and I will use it the way I please."

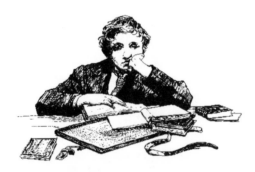

Indifference to education is a variant of indifference to work, and, here again, the ubiquitous *Sulphur* is among the leaders—once more exhibiting a characteristic that is the polar opposite of his usual passion for study and education.

We recall that *Sulphur,* the quintessential scholar, pedagogue, philosopher (genuine or false), and truth-seeker, loves to amass facts and information. He can regale a captive audience with an eloquent disquisition on the anatomical structure of the 650 sub-species of mosquito, or with detailed and exhaustive explanations of the Urdu or Chinese roots of words like "polo" or "tea" for hours on end; but he can also disdain learning and be truly indifferent to its value and importance (see the chapter on *Sulphur*).

This is one reason why *Sulphur* is so often the simillimum for the formerly curious and intellectually eager adolescent who has now rebelled and become resolutely indifferent to his studies.

Calcarea carbonica manifests a similar indifference but without *Sulphur*'s disdain. He simply does not "feel like" continuing his education—a symptom which fits Kent's "indifference to important things" (where *Calcarea* is one of only two remedies listed). This trait often reflects *Calcarea*'s native indolence and lack of ambition.

An intelligent college student, who considered himself knowledgeable enough to succeed in life without further education, used his chronic nasal catarrh and sinus pain as an excuse to quit school. His decision was not due to restlessness or inability to concentrate, to physical weakness or fatigue, but merely to apathy: he was not really satisfied by anything college had offered him so far.

All his physical symptoms fitted *Calcarea* and were greatly alleviated by this remedy, but his lack of motivation was unaffected. The mindset of a resistant *Calcarea* is well-known to be difficult to alter once physical growth and development have ceased. If the remedy had been prescribed earlier, in his formative years, the outcome might well have been different.

In contrast to *Calcarea,* the indifference of *Lachesis* to education carries a rebellious note and is often the reflection of some powerful underlying feeling. An example is the boy of sixteen who was being treated for a tendency to truancy; while exceptionally intelligent, he was failing his courses and totally lacked any sense of responsibility. He was not anti-intellectual but refused to study and wasted his own and others' time being the class joker. His sharp tongue and oft-professed indifference to the need for a high-school diploma (using ridicule to justify his own indifference to it) were very *Lachesis.*

While physically healthy and symptom-free, he was *Lachesis* in other respects, exhibiting the type's bright darting eye as well as its suspicious nature. "I don't want you to give me snake poison or anything like that," he protested, before the physician had even resolved on the remedy. And, after receiving the medicine under his tongue, he promptly tried to spit out the (fortunately!) rapidly dissolving granules.

For several ensuing weeks there was no sign that his papers would be handed in on time, or that his attitude would change. But one morning he awoke and, setting aside his rebellious proclivities, resolved to apply himself to the books. "I don't know why I made that decision," he said. "It was like suddenly deciding to give up smoking."

This was his only explanation of the subtle action of *Lachesis* on his psyche.

The patient needing *Phosphoric acid* usually becomes indifferent to studies because of external factors: difficulties in relationships, exhaustion from stress, overwork, or a previous illness. There is no lack of interest *per se,* no principled stance or ideological protest, nor is this indifference innate to the type. He simply does not have the emotional strength to continue with his studies ("mental enfeeblement": Kent).

Typical here was the young woman, happy in graduate school, who, after a series of bouts of influenza, could not be motivated to resume her studies. "I am suffering from erosion of memory and dimming of the imagination," she would maintain. "Any structured thinking makes me giddy."

This was a close approximation of Hahnemann's "weakness of mind; on reflecting he becomes dizzy. Indolent dull mind without elasticity, no imagination . . . he cannot get his ideas into their proper connection," but the physician only discovered this later.

Meanwhile, several remedies were prescribed, but to no avail. A striking, and therefore guiding, symptom was that, despite her feebleness, she looked deceptively well. *Phosphoric acid,* like *Phosphorus,* fits this characteristic ("he does not look actually ill": Hahnemann) and was the remedy that finally motivated her to get on with her life.

Indifference to Social Conventions and Amenities

Indifference to social conventions and amenities, to accepted manners, is an elusive trait, since it has little to do with reason or logic yet is often stronger than both of these. It is a challenge to the unspoken assumptions that underlie the social culture.

Free-spirited indifference to the prevailing norms of behavior is not uncommon in young persons of various constitutional types, but when this attitude persists into adulthood, the patient manifesting chronically unconventional deportment, certain typical remedy pictures emerge: most prominently *Natrum muriaticum, Lachesis, Sulphur,* and, to a lesser degree, *Phosphoric acid.*

The *Phosphoric acid* individual who behaves oddly is usually the victim of some emotional trauma. He is quiet and withdrawn, polite enough, and even apparently attentive and considerate, but in reality he is abstracted, and his thoughts are elsewhere. He is oblivious to the world's opinion because he is engrossed in his own preoccupations. The run-of-the-mill problems that concern others leave him unperturbed. He shuts himself off from those who have not passed through the same trauma and becomes indifferent to conventional values.

Ruthie Stone, the sensitive and deeply injured young protagonist of Marilynne Robinson's book, *Housekeeping,* suffering from the "chronic effects of fright" (Hering) after her mother's suicide, is a literary example of this type. As she takes on the eccentric behavior and mannerisms of her itinerant aunt, she is propelled onto a different plane where she is no longer sensitive to the traditional amenities.

Natrum muriaticum is somewhat different. He tries repeatedly without success to gain acceptance of his naturally quirky personality; he then tries, and again fails, to mold his character according to others' expectations; finally he decides, or is compelled, to abandon the striving and resigns himself to his odd or different manner and a growing estrangement from society, and sometimes even family.

Manners, after all, by expressing implied social and cultural values, draw people together, or separate them, more strongly, perhaps, than even religion, politics, or morals.

Furthermore, however sincere his efforts to adapt to the prevailing norm, and despite all pressures to the contrary from his peers or from society, *Natrum muriaticum* remains doggedly true to his own idiosyncratic self. And once settled into this defiant mode, he easily takes on a tone of self-righteous superiority and grows increasingly indifferent to the ordinary conventions and assumptions. It then becomes harder and harder to return to "normalcy."

The idiosyncratic *Natrum muriaticum* symptom, "indifferent when in society" (Kent), is not just reluctance to open up a chink in his protective armor and expose his vulnerability to strangers. Nor is it mere unwillingness to participate in a group where he cannot dominate. It is just that in these circumstances he has absolutely nothing to say!

With close friends, and especially in tête-a-tête conversations, where all parties speak truthfully and sincerely, he can be the liveliest of interlocutors. But in a larger group he is, rightly or wrongly, sensitive to the vapidity of the conversation and the falsity of the group dynamics. He finds that subtle ideas are oversimplified; that emotions, once verbalized, become false; that delicate feelings become crude and profound ones superficial or egoistic; that all meanings are woefully perverted or distorted.

But his "indifference when in society" is a far cry from unresponsiveness *toward* society. His seeming apathy masks a powerful compassion for humanity in general or, not to put too fine a point on it, an obsession with social injustice and inequity. Seeking recogni-

tion of his nobility and righteousness (which, because of his uncon-
ventionality, he has difficulty obtaining) he remains, even when per-
sonally estranged, ever sensitive to the social order, ever anxious
to guide the world to "rightness." His hand reaches out to help,
and when he cannot help, in his disillusionment he may turn de-
spondent, but not indifferent.

Lachesis also finds an outlet in contorted or erratic behavior
when unable to adapt to accepted norms. Despite repeated assur-
ances of love for life and enjoyment of it, his history often reveals
a long run of "bad luck," a series of mishaps, suggesting that his
spirit has been in some impalpable way broken, leaving him with
a protective coat of estrangement from, and indifference to, the
prevailing social mores.

He is not subdued by hardship but is rather propelled into a
higher state of energy, a manic transport of feeling, with growing
imperviousness to the stigma of eccentricity.

One such patient was the woman who suffered from the wonder-
fully "strange, rare, and peculiar" symptom of a daily swelling of the
left breast and, indeed, the left side of the chest and upper left arm.
The heart itself felt swollen, she maintained ("heart, as if swelled":
Boger), and she often awoke at night with a feeling of suffocation,
as if some furry animal was nestling on her chest just under her chin.*
She was greatly helped by *Lachesis* after allopathic medicine had
been unable to assist her in any way or, indeed, even to diagnose
her condition.

Just as "strange, rare, and peculiar" were the workings of her
mind. One day, in a transport of gratitude to the physician who,

---

*Fortunately, the furry animal was benign—like a "friendly kitty-
cat," as the patient said. In two other such cases known to the
author (both *Lachesis*) the furry objects lodging on the chest were
malign (the male patient wrestled with a succubus, the female with
an incubus).

she felt, had saved her sanity, if not her life, she exclaimed, "I'm so thankful for all you've done that I would like to die for you!"

"No, please," the physician remonstrated. "This would just undo all our good work."

"All right," she replied, only slightly deflated at having her proffered sacrifice so promptly rejected, "then I'll make you a blueberry pie instead."

The physician gratefully accepted this latter alternative.

Yet another female patient, with a left-sided facial neuralgia of long standing, who realized she was considered peculiar but was indifferent to it, volunteered in explanation: "What do I care for conventional mores and amenities? For forty years I was a law-abiding church-going citizen, but life has so consistently demonstrated to me that no *good* deed goes unpunished, no effort to adapt to accepted modes of behavior is recognized, that I finally decided against striving for acceptance on others' terms. Now I act as I please, in *total* disregard of public opinion."

The physician sensed the truth of her observations. In fact, as a homoeopath on the fringes of the medically acceptable, he could even sympathize with them. But her cavalier disregard of society's norms took its toll. By acting willfully and erratically this *Lachesis* set herself apart from others and paid a price in isolation and estrangement.

It took many months of homoeopathic treatment, primarily with *Lachesis* 5M as a constitutional remedy, to cure the patient of her symptoms and enable her to find a balance between indifference to society's demands and respect for them.

Sulphur's indifference to social expectations is rooted in *refusal* to be influenced or modified, to compromise by even one iota his particular stance or conviction.

Lycopodium may be equally self-righteous but is seldom equally indifferent to what is expected of him. He is respectful of social expectations.

Indifference in either of these does not necessarily mean lack of social awareness or an exploitative attitude. Both simply hold the conviction that "What benefits me benefits the entire world!" and expect the entire world to adjust accordingly.

All of the constitutional types discussed in this section may affect moral superiority. Once they have set foot on the unconventional path and experienced the heady feeling of being unencumbered by social strictures and assumptions, once they have risen above the mundane concerns and trivia of ordinary life, they tend to disparage any other mode of behavior.

Indifference to conventions and manners, however, must be distinguished from indifference to standards of morality. Criminal or sociopathic behavior is a separate issue that lies beyond the subject matter and scope of this chapter.

A specific form of indifference to others' opinions is "indifference to personal appearance" (Kent).

The rebel has always proclaimed his conflict with society by neglecting his dress and appearance. While *Sulphur* is the only remedy listed under this rubric by Kent, several others could also be mentioned.

Sulphur's disregard of appearances (like his indifference to pleasure) is often rooted in a principled challenge to "decadent bourgeois values." If he were to cut his hair or dress with elegance, his appearance would not harmonize with his high-minded principles, his outer being would be out of step with his inner self, and *Sulphur* refuses to participate in such a gross deception.

His self-absorbed egocentrism also plays a role. Wrapped in his private thoughts, he becomes oblivious to his surroundings—to the (in his eyes) specious and superficial manifestations of the world (the remedy, we recall, is also listed by Kent under "indifference to external things"). His mismatched socks or missing shirt buttons might reflect absent-mindedness, but his unkempt dishevelled appearance proceeds from unconcern for others.

He does not have to look at himself. *He* is not offended by his own aroma. So why should he be concerned with cleanliness or tidiness? The type, moreover, is characteristically reluctant to let go of any part of himself (i.e., hair, article of clothing), and the whole is compounded by a subliminal streak of miserliness. Bathing uses up soap and hot water; shaving uses up razor blades (which he hates to discard) and consumes electricity (which he must pay for); washing clothes wears them out prematurely, and so forth. One *Sulphur* husband regarded his wife's every attempt to put his dirty clothes in the wash as an assault upon his dignity. When she spirited them away at night under cover of darkness, he would awaken and cry out in mock despair tinged with genuine irritation, "Why are you taking away my clothes before they are really dirty? It's like burying me before I'm dead."

Sometimes the *Sulphur* man who looks like a hobo, or the woman who resembles a "bag lady," exhibits meticulous care in some particular field of endeavor ("revolving neglect," as one patient expressed it). Concern with appearances, they argue, would only detract from their true mission in life.

Calcarea carbonica's disregard of personal appearance reflects, as always, his native indolence. Anyway he prefers comfort to looks, meaning loose formless garb, suspenders instead of a belt (he cannot tolerate constriction around the waist or abdomen; also *Lycopodium*), floppy shoes and hats, and so on.

In addition, because he has trouble getting down to work, especially when at home, and is easily distracted by petty unimportant concerns, merely putting on his clothes in the morning can ruin his concentration for the rest of the day. Thus one readily finds him— at any hour of the twenty-four—working in bathrobe or pyjamas. When queried about this, he will cite such famous writers as Samuel Johnson, Pushkin, or Balzac who, according to him, could only write in their dressing gowns (perhaps they, too, had much *Calcarea carbonica* in their constitutional economy).

The disregard for appearances extends to the home. *Sulphur* and *Calcarea* do not pick up after themselves. The desk is covered with rings from innumerable cups and glasses; the cups themselves are stained with ink, the glasses with grease. A plate from last week's dinner, accommodating a shrivelled and now unidentifiable morsel, is used as a paperweight or perched on a stack of books. Dirty dishes are piled in the sink, and stacks of old newspapers, grocery bags, empty bottles, and the like litter the premises.

In *Sulphur* this reflects the "collector" mentality. In *Calcarea carbonica* hanging on to useless objects can often be traced back to a traumatic loss. Having already been deprived of much in life, he is now reluctant to relinquish anything.

True, the *Calcarea* woman will sometimes pick up for guests, out of guilt or pride of home, rushing around frantically to make her house presentable when warned of their coming. But if they then fail to appear, she grumbles resentfully, "What a waste! Like a fool I cleaned up my house all for nothing."

Natrum muriaticum can also be indifferent to dress. Oddly, this type is actually quite self-conscious about her appearance but, as in so much else, entirely perverse. If, for reasons of size, shape, facial features, or lack of finances, she cannot satisfy her own, often peculiar, standards of sartorial elegance, she goes to the other extreme and puts on whatever is handy. Or she may just scorn indulgence in these vanities where so many existential problems remain to be resolved; the hair in disarray, unfashionable clothes, and neglected home are thus deliberate statements of protest. Believing with *Sulphur* that appearances should truthfully reflect the inner being, she considers that stylish dress or coiffure ill become an individual who is so conscious of with the deplorable state of the world.

Phosphoric acid may also be indifferent to the appearance of his home or person, but it is a temporary aberration, resulting from illness, shock, or emotional trauma. It is neither as chronic and long-lasting as the indifference of *Sulphur* or *Calcarea,* nor as principled and consistent as that of *Natrum muriaticum.* Nor, in contrast to *Lachesis,* does disarray of dress and grooming reflect mental agitation, inner turmoil, or a disturbed and chaotic psyche.

Indifference to Affection and to Attachments

Finally, we take up indifference to affection and attachments ("indifference to loved ones": Kent), which may be the most common manifestation of this mental state.

Relations with others and expectations of them inevitably entail some pain and disillusionment. Everyone cultivates some degree of indifference which, like a moat around the fortress of the heart, wards off the traumas of loss and disappointment.

Phosphoric acid is a major remedy for patients who, in self defense, attempt to barricade *all* access to deeper emotional attachments.

One middle-aged woman treated for arthritic pains and alarming loss of hair (it was falling out in handfuls—a key symptom of *Phosphoric acid*) had long been in a stressful marriage and had been severely disappointed in her two adopted children. Having experienced the instability of human affections and despairing of satisfaction from any close relationship, she had turned indifferent to her family and friends and gone off to live on her own.

Asked if she were lonely, she replied, "Yes, at first, but then you get used to it and do not mind the solitude. At least you are not torn apart by pain, doubt, and false expectations. Eventually you cease to care about those who have hurt you, and, with time, it becomes hard to imagine one's life as other than lonely and detached. I now accept it as a natural form of existence and don't wish for anything different."

Phosphoric acid exhibits little sympathy for Tennyson's "'Tis better to have loved and lost than never to have loved at all." Far better, she believes, never to have loved at all than to have suffered as she has suffered. In contrast to the high romanticism of *Phosphorus, Tuberculinum,* or *Ignatia,* who will sacrifice peace of mind for moments of rapture and insist that, despite the pain and grief they have endured, they would not have foregone this particular love for anything, *Phosphoric acid* welcomes a *soothing* indifference.

The physician was wary of intruding on this stabilizing indifference. When caring entails so much pain, the defense mechanism should not be disturbed. Yet the patient's body was obviously at odds with this new psychic mode and refused to condone her emotional emptiness.

Her physical health was restored, without jeopardizing her still fragile healing indifference, by several doses of *Phosphoric acid* in *medium* potency (30C; a higher potency might just have aggravated her mental picture). A viable balance between body and mind had apparently been established.

Another female patient presenting the *Phosphoric acid* indifference of the affections, who had suffered for fifteen years from a debilitating cough, was cured overnight by a does of this remedy. Her ailment had started after a failed love affair. Ever since, she had been indifferent to romantic attachments—cutting off, as it were, that side of her emotional life, and pushing it into a far corner of her mind. Here the physician wanted to act on a long standing emotional state, so he prescribed *Phosphoric acid* in the 10M potency. It did dispose of the cough, but the patient left town shortly thereafter, and her subsequent emotional development is unknown.

Ignatia's emotional indifference is less permanent than that of *Phosphoric acid;* usually the patient is prepared to respond and feel again at the first opportunity (see the *Ignatia* chapter). But it is sometimes hard to distinguish between the two, and the choice may depend on the concomitant physical symptoms, general modalities, or, if the physician is lucky, some "strange, rare, and peculiar" symptom. The two following animal cases illustrate this.

The first was a short-haired black mutt whose owners had moved and left her with neighbors. She resembled a cross between a Labrador retriever and a chihuahua, with a bushy squirrel-like tail that stuck straight up and a porcine snout (if such an ungainly blend can be imagined). But most striking was her personality. Running free in her semi-rural environment, she displayed the ceaseless erratic energy and purposeless movements of a buzzing fly. Sometimes she ran around in circles from the sheer joy of existence, and she also had a talent for stirring up the other neighborhood dogs with her high pitched yapping and teasing manner.

This little creature now became completely apathetic, her formerly bright protruding eyes lusterless and sunken. She was indifferent to food, rejected affection, and refused to go outside and cavort with her buddies. Instead she lay all day on the hearth by the fireplace.

Her formerly "active, lively, cheerful disposition" and her doggish variation on the guiding symptom, "dejected when walking in open air, in the house . . . becomes more cheerful" (Hahnemann), pointed to a prescription of *Phosphoric acid* rather than *Ignatia*.

After a couple of days she had so completely recovered her former spirits, and so increased the noise level in the neighborhood, that her new owners somewhat regretted that the medicine had worked so well.

The second case was a baby raccoon, three or four weeks old, washed out of his nest by a violent thunderstorm, and brought by a state trooper to the home of an animal lover. Obviously pining for his mother, he refused all food and milk, and his survival was despaired of until *Ignatia* 200X was prescribed—daily for three days.

Here, again, the remedy proved almost too effective. The animal thrived and became a menace to the household. With his dexterous human-like hands he opened drawers and closets, tore up bills and letters, napped in the electric blender by day and in the baby's crib at night. Finally he had to be given away to a children's zoo, where he entertained a wider audience with his captivating antics and engaging personality.

The nagging question always remains: if the remedies received by these two animals had been interchanged, would the results have been as gratifying?

Since every case is unique, an unambiguous answer cannot be given. But experience suggests that a patient often can be bene-fitted by more than one remedy, at a given point in time.

Of course there can be only one *simillimum,* since only one remedy can be "the *most* similar." But God is merciful, and other remedies, while only "similars" *(similes),* can still be of assistance. Presumably, each affects a slightly different aspect of the body-mind complex—resonates at a different level, so to speak—in the curative process. *

The *Phosphorus* indifference to affection, listed by Kent vari-ously as "indifference to loved ones . . . to relations . . . to his chil-dren," carries its own particular aura of flightiness, instability, or superficiality.

This incapacity to feel contrasts with the type's usual warmth, affection, and sensitivity to the needs of others. The person *who used to ingratiate* by his emotional responsiveness no longer cares whether he is pleasing or not. As if wearied of being bright, cheer-ful, and reactive, he seeks to escape this responsibility. His grace and charm which had always drawn others into his circle are now imposing too heavy demands on his personality.

The indifference of *Phosphorus* is thus acquired, not innate, and defined primarily by that which it negates: the need for com-panionship, the fear of loneliness, and, indeed, his own self-love.

Lycopodium, in contrast, exhibits a truer indifference to the af-fections, one inherent to his constitutional makeup and which is the natural corollary of his detachment.

On one level he values friendship, respects family ties, and believes in marriage. Yet time and again one hears a *Lycopodium*

---

*These broader questions of method are discussed in the *Silica* and *Staphysagria* chapters and in the Conclusion of *Portraits,* vol. 2.

patient say of his marriage: "I like my wife, respect her, and wish
her well. But she, simply, is not essential to my happiness." But then,
no one really is. He easily weathers the rupture of close relationships, despite the social graces he exerts to disguise this fact from
himself and others. After all, his conscious and unconscious emotional life is largely devoted to avoiding *binding* attachments that
have the potential of becoming troublesome or too close contact
with his deeper feelings. Thus, after the initial inconvenience or un-
pleasantness, he finds himself ultimately indifferent to the rupture—
indeed relieved that the emotionally demanding relationship has
ended (see chapter on *Lycopodium*).

But, to give *Lycopodium* his due, his genuine indifference to
deep attachments is not calculated selfishness, callousness, or con-
tempt for these relationships. He may even be distressed by his own
attitude. But he strives instinctively to remain uncommitted. That
is why, unless he makes a conscious effort to combat this tendency,
he lets those closest to him subtly understand that he hardly feels
more for them than for any casual acquaintance, for his work, his
travels, or his splendid book or record collection.

Arsenicum is less subtle. He may be polite, but his "indifference
and lack of sympathy" (Hahnemann) are clearly felt in his tone of
voice.

Sulphur's indifference to affection is suggested by Kent's listing
it under "indifference to the welfare of others" (the only remedy
so honored). This is an injustice to other medicines displaying this
characteristic, but *Sulphur* is certainly more forthright and conceals
neither his positive nor his negative qualities. Like a volcano in erup-
tion, everything in him rises to the surface and is there for all to
see (we recall how his physical and emotional ailments often come
out on the skin).

Otherwise his indifference to close attachments is more like that
of *Lycopodium*—due to preoccupation with his work, hobbies, or
other interests. Or it reflects self-absorption and consequent inability

to appreciate another's viewpoint.

One writer who loved above all else to reread his own writings declared, only half jokingly, "Frankly, I become bored after ten minutes when left in the society of any other author but myself."

But *Sepia* is the front runner in the indifference-to-affection contest. Usually her apathy is due to physical lethargy—a prostration so complete that even the pretence of caring becomes burdensome.

The *Sepia* woman's standoffishness in familial and romantic love ("indifferent to those she loves best": Hering) has been discussed thoroughly in that chapter. Suffice it here to note that, although her sexual indifference can sometimes be genuine, her apparent apathy can also be a strategic ploy.

She is not dull-witted and realizes quite well that apparent aloofness or detachment has a powerful attraction for the opposite sex. Indeed, many men seem to prefer their women cold (see Ring Lardner's semi-comic rendering of this theme in his short-story, "Some Like 'Em Cold"). Modelling her indifference on that of the *Lycopodium* male (whose emotional elusiveness is one of the clues to his sexual attraction), she cultivates it not only for self-protection but also for power over the other.

A clever and attractive woman suffering from incapacitatingly painful menstrual cramps was recognized as needing *Sepia* when she volunteered, "Men were not interested in me when I was warm and responsive, and would even shy away. Now that I pretend indifference or act careless—sometimes even arrogant, they are appreciative. Perhaps they are attracted by what they judge to be strength, or perhaps they see my inaccessibility as an interesting challenge—who knows? But my aloofness is now becoming second nature, and I really do feel indifference about most people. While I don't want to become hard, I cannot afford to relinquish my indifference and become vulnerable again."

This dilemma, and the menstrual cramps, were resolved to the patient's satisfaction by *Sepia* 10M.

All in all, this type learns more easily than *Natrum muriaticum, Staphysagria, Ignatia,* or *Phosphorus* that in relationships one must often hold back emotionally so as to give others a chance to take the initiative. A perpetually giving nature is liable to be taken for granted, while distance and indifference breed appreciation and respect.

This strategy, of course, does not hold true for young children, but *Sepia* can, mistakenly or unconsciously, even be "indifferent to her children" (Kent).

Sometimes her seeming lack of care or feeling is really a dispassionate judgment. A patient experiencing severe menopausal hot flashes together with a deteriorating marriage was prescribed this remedy with success partly on the basis of her strangely unperturbed response to the impending separation. "Of course I am sad to see my twenty-five year marriage dissolve, for I love my husband, and this is entirely his decision. But, on the other hand, I have observed that women grow more through disappointment in love than through any other experience. This may be the only way to prod them out of their psychological stasis into the new roles they will have to assume in the latter years of the twentieth century—the only way to force them to discover their talents and potential and decide how to contribute to the survival of this planet. So (with a shrug of indifference that dispelled self-pity) why should I be exempt from this opportunity for growth?"

Natrum muriaticum's and *Staphysagria*'s indifference to affection arises almost invariably out of reaction to emotional injury. Since the harvest of pain these two types can reap from wounds to their affections consistently surpasses even their own expectations in richness and abundance, they learn to take measures to forestall the next bountiful crop. To exchange sorrow for a "sweet indifference," as the nineteenth-century Romantic poets liked to call it, is thus a virtual liberation.

But the quiescent surface conceals intense and vigorously sustained emotional activity.

A case illustrating *Natrum muriaticum*'s prodigious capacity for holding grudges, disguised as lack of interest, was the man of forty who sought homoeopathic assistance for an unhappy mental state. Questioning revealed that he had left his family at age eighteen and for more than twenty years had had almost no contact with them. This had been provoked by the shattering discovery that his mother, who was unhappy in her marriage, was having love affairs. He had been enraged for several years after finding this out but then completely lost interest in her well-being and remained in that state for almost two decades. But there was still much smoldering resentment. "I have cultivated indifference," he admitted, "but quite honestly I still long to hit her."

Half a dozen doses of *Natrum muriaticum* 50M were required over the next year, spelled occasionally by *Staphysagria* 50M, to induce this sadly bruised and misguided idealist to relinquish his moral rigidity and venture out of his unhealthy indifference. Only after this intense treatment was he willing again to risk his affections with his parents—who, for their part, warmly welcomed back their Prodigal Son.*

At times *Natrum muriaticum* and *Staphysagria* patients admit to feigning indifference while, in reality, *longing for emotional attachment without penalty or disillusionment.* But when destiny does not vouchsafe them this gift, or when possession does little to satisfy love's yearning, they cultivate a *pose* of indifference.

Yet in these *Natrum muriaticum* or *Staphysagria* instances, as in other cases of psychic injury, often the patient need only

---

*But *Natrum muriaticum*'s relations with his (or her) offspring are often an exception. Having suffered so much from his own parents, he is extra sensitive to the emotional needs of his children and relates well to them.

acknowledge an emotion, and the painful process of dredging up and analyzing the subconscious can be circumvented.

In its beautiful simplicity and capacity to *cut through* (rather than unravel) the tangle of the ever-mysterious mind-body complex, homoeopathy reminds us of those fairy tales of the Brothers Grimm in which the simple solution succeeds where learned explanations and complicated devices have been unavailing. The princess who cannot cry over the most unfortunate event is cured by peeling an onion; the young man who cannot shiver or shudder, despite elaborate attempts to frighten him, finally does so when his bed is doused with cold water from the stream (together with its wriggling minnows), and so forth.

Such is the healing power of the simillimum.

The Healthy Indifference

In conclusion we would repeat that no sensitive physician would dispossess a patient of his hard-earned protective (even though sometimes only skin deep) indifference. His approach in helping to cherish this precious acquisition must be delicate and gingerly.

"Healthy" indifference is a matter of balance. One that conceals apathy, idleness, lack of interest, and self-inflicted denial is, certainly, inferior to vital feelings or caring relationships. But for some morbidly sensitive and excessively vulnerable individuals such an indifference may be more than desirable—it is a necessity. It restores self-respect by encouraging the stoicism and reserve that arise out of a principled refusal to experience more painful emotion than the situation demands. It also acts as an intermediate balancing stage in the psyche's passage from pain to relief.

In this function, indifference can be viewed as a healthy transition from anguished despair to the calm acceptance which signifies cure.

FREQUENCY OF REMEDIES USED FOR INDIFFERENCE

GENUINE

MASKING

CARBO VEGETABILIS

Gelsemium

Psorinum

Opium

PHOSPHORIC ACID

SEPIA

Sulphur

Calcarea carbonica

Lycopodium

Pulsatilla

NATRUM MURIATICUM

Staphysagria

Ignatia

Arsenicum album